The Essential Foods Lists For Kidney Disease

Nourishing Recipes and Dietary Strategies
for Managing Kidney Disease

McDonnell B. Young

Table of Contents

Introduction

Emma had always been the rock of her family—juggling her demanding job, caring for her two young children, and still finding time to volunteer at the local community center. But when she was diagnosed with early-stage kidney disease, everything changed. The news was overwhelming, and her once carefully balanced life seemed to crumble.

Her doctor explained that diet would play a crucial role in managing her condition. Emma was handed a stack of pamphlets and a vague list of foods to avoid, but nothing seemed to offer the comprehensive guidance she needed. Frustrated and confused, she turned to the internet, only to find conflicting advice and complicated medical jargon. She felt lost and helpless.

One evening, while scrolling through her social media feed, Emma came across a post about a new guide called "The Essential Foods Lists For Kidney Disease." The title caught her attention immediately. The post promised a clear, detailed, and comprehensive approach to managing kidney disease through diet. Intrigued, she clicked on the link and started reading reviews from others who had used the guide.

One review stood out. It was from a mother who described how the guide had transformed her life. She shared how easy it was to follow, how it demystified what foods were beneficial and which to avoid, and how it offered practical tips for meal planning and preparation. The guide had become her go-to resource, helping her regain control of her health and improve her quality of life.

Emma felt a glimmer of hope. She decided to purchase "The Essential Foods Lists For Kidney Disease." When the guide arrived, she was immediately impressed by its structure. The introduction explained kidney disease in simple terms and highlighted the critical role of diet in managing the condition. It felt like a friend was gently guiding her through the maze of dietary choices.

As she delved deeper into the book, Emma discovered detailed lists of foods to eat and foods to avoid, complete with explanations of why each food was included. The guide didn't just tell her what to eat; it explained how to prepare meals, offered delicious recipes, and provided tips for dining out and managing cravings. The sections on reading food labels and portion control were particularly enlightening. She realized how many hidden dangers she had been unaware of in her previous diet.

One Saturday morning, armed with her new knowledge, Emma went grocery shopping. For the first time in months, she felt confident about her choices. She filled her cart with kidney-friendly foods like fresh vegetables, lean proteins, and low-potassium fruits. At home, she prepared a meal from one of the guide's recipes—a grilled chicken with a vibrant vegetable medley. Her family loved it, and Emma felt a sense of accomplishment and relief.

Over the following weeks, Emma noticed significant improvements in her health and energy levels. She no longer felt the constant fatigue that had plagued her since her diagnosis. Her doctor was pleased with her progress and commended her efforts in adhering to a kidney-friendly diet. Emma even found that her new way of eating benefited her entire family, promoting overall health and well-being.

"The Essential Foods Lists For Kidney Disease" became Emma's trusted companion. It sat on her kitchen counter, dog-eared and annotated, a testament to her journey toward better health. She recommended it to friends and even shared it with her local support group, hoping it would help others as much as it had helped her.

In a world where navigating dietary restrictions can feel like an impossible task, "The Essential Foods Lists For Kidney Disease" provided Emma with clarity, support, and hope. It was more than just a guide; it was a lifeline. For anyone facing the challenges of kidney disease, this book was not just a purchase—it was an investment in their health and future.

Understanding Kidney Disease

Kidney disease is a condition that affects the kidneys' ability to filter waste and excess fluids from the blood, which can lead to the accumulation of toxins in the body. This condition can be chronic, developing slowly over time, or acute, occurring suddenly due to injury or illness. Managing kidney disease often requires a multifaceted approach, with diet playing a crucial role. When dealing with kidney disease, it's essential to understand how certain foods can impact kidney function and overall health.

The kidneys are responsible for balancing electrolytes, maintaining blood pressure, and producing hormones that regulate red blood cell production and bone health. When they are compromised, these functions can be disrupted, leading to various health issues. High levels of certain minerals, such as potassium, phosphorus, and sodium, can be particularly harmful to individuals with kidney disease. Therefore, understanding which foods contain these minerals and how they affect the kidneys is vital for managing the condition.

A diet tailored to kidney disease focuses on controlling the intake of potassium, phosphorus, and sodium to prevent further kidney damage and alleviate symptoms. Potassium is necessary for muscle function and heart health, but high levels can be dangerous for those with kidney disease. Foods such as bananas, oranges, and potatoes are high in potassium and may need to be limited or avoided. On the other hand, low-potassium options like apples, berries, and cabbage can be included in the diet.

Phosphorus is another mineral that needs to be managed carefully. It helps in bone formation and energy storage, but excess phosphorus can lead to bone and heart problems in individuals with kidney disease. Foods high in phosphorus, such as dairy products, nuts, and seeds, should be consumed in moderation. Alternatives like rice milk and certain fruits and vegetables can help maintain a balanced diet without overloading the kidneys with phosphorus.

Sodium control is also critical, as high sodium intake can increase blood pressure and exacerbate kidney disease symptoms. Processed foods, canned soups, and fast foods are typically high in sodium and should be minimized. Instead, fresh, unprocessed foods and herbs can be used to flavor meals without adding extra sodium. Learning to read food labels and understanding the sodium content of different foods can aid in making healthier choices.

In addition to managing these key minerals, protein intake must be monitored. While protein is essential for body repair and growth, excessive amounts can strain the kidneys. Individuals with kidney disease often need to balance their protein intake by choosing high-quality protein sources, such as lean meats, fish, and egg whites, and incorporating plant-based proteins in moderation.

Hydration is another critical aspect of managing kidney disease. Proper fluid intake helps the kidneys flush out toxins, but the amount of fluid needed can vary depending on the stage of the disease and individual health conditions. Consulting with a healthcare provider to determine the right balance is crucial. Drinking plenty of water and choosing beverages low in sugar and additives can support kidney health.

Understanding kidney disease and its dietary implications is essential for effective management. "The Essential Foods Lists For Kidney Disease" provides a comprehensive guide to navigating these dietary restrictions, offering clear information on which foods to eat and which to avoid. By following the guidelines in this book, individuals can take control of their diet, support their kidney function, and improve their overall quality of life.

Chapter 1: Foods to Eat for Kidney Disease

Vegetables

Here's a detailed table covering 15 vegetables suitable for a kidney-friendly diet, including their ingredients, instructions, nutritional information, serving size, and cooking time.

Vegetable	Ingredients	Instructions	Nutritional Information (per 1 cup cooked)	Serving Size	Cooking Time
Cabbage	Fresh cabbage leaves	Chop cabbage, steam or sauté until tender.	33 calories, 1.4g protein, 0.1g fat, 7.6g carbs,	1 cup	5-7 minutes (steamed)

			1.2g fiber, 126mg potassium		
Caulifl ower	Fresh cauliflo wer florets	Cut into florets, steam or roast until tender.	25 calories, 2g protein, 0.1g fat, 5g carbs, 2g fiber, 176mg potassium	1 cup	5-10 minutes (steame d)
Bell Pepper s	Fresh bell peppers (any color)	Slice and grill or sauté until tender.	30 calories, 1g protein, 0.2g fat, 7g carbs, 2.5g fiber,	1 cup	5-7 minutes (sautée d)

			261mg potassium		
Zucchini	Fresh zucchini	Slice and sauté or grill until tender.	33 calories, 2.4g protein, 0.6g fat, 6g carbs, 2g fiber, 295mg potassium	1 cup	5-7 minutes (sautéed)
Green Beans	Fresh green beans	Trim ends, steam or sauté until tender.	44 calories, 2g protein, 0.3g fat, 10g carbs, 4g fiber, 180mg potassium	1 cup	5-7 minutes (steamed)

Aspara gus	Fresh asparag us spears	Trim ends, steam or grill until tender.	20 calories, 2.2g protein, 0.2g fat, 4g carbs, 2g fiber, 202mg potassi um	1 cup	5-7 minutes (steame d)
Spinac h (cooke d)	Fresh spinach leaves	Wash and cook until wilted.	41 calories, 5g protein, 0.5g fat, 7g carbs, 4g fiber, 840mg potassi um	1 cup	3-4 minutes (steame d)
Brussel s	Fresh Brussels sprouts	Trim and cut in half,	38 calories, 3g	1 cup	6-8 minutes

Sprouts		steam or roast until tender.	protein, 0.3g fat, 8g carbs, 3g fiber, 342mg potassium		(steamed)
Carrots	Fresh carrots	Peel and slice, steam or roast until tender.	55 calories, 1.2g protein, 0.3g fat, 13g carbs, 3.5g fiber, 390mg potassium	1 cup	5-7 minutes (steamed)
Butternut Squash	Fresh butternut squash, peeled	Peel, cube, and roast	82 calories, 1.8g protein, 0.2g fat,	1 cup	20-25 minutes (roasted)

	and cubed	until tender.	22g carbs, 6g fiber, 582mg potassium		
Tomatoes	Fresh tomatoes (for cooking)	Chop and cook in sauce or soup.	32 calories, 1.5g protein, 0.4g fat, 7g carbs, 2g fiber, 427mg potassium	1 cup	10-15 minutes (cooked)
Beetroot	Fresh beetroot, peeled and cubed	Boil or roast until tender.	58 calories, 2.2g protein, 0.2g fat, 13g carbs, 4g fiber,	1 cup	30-40 minutes (boiled)

			305mg potassium		
Kale	Fresh kale leaves	Wash and sauté or steam until wilted.	36 calories, 2.5g protein, 0.5g fat, 7g carbs, 1.3g fiber, 296mg potassium	1 cup	5-7 minutes (steamed)
Collard Greens	Fresh collard greens	Wash and cook until tender.	63 calories, 5g protein, 1g fat, 11g carbs, 5g fiber, 400mg	1 cup	15-20 minutes (steamed)

			potassium		
Celery	Fresh celery stalks	Slice and eat raw or cook in soups and stews.	16 calories, 0.7g protein, 0.2g fat, 3g carbs, 1.6g fiber, 260mg potassium	1 cup	5 minutes (steamed)

This table provides a range of kidney-friendly vegetables, including instructions for preparation, nutritional information to help manage mineral intake, and cooking times to aid in meal planning.

Fruits

Here's a detailed table about fruits that are suitable for individuals with kidney disease, including ingredient information, instructions, nutritional details, serving size, and preparation time:

Fruit	Ingredient	Instructions	Nutritional Information	Serving Size	Preparation Time
Apples	Fresh apples	Wash thoroughly. Slice and remove seeds. Can be eaten raw or cooked.	Calories: 95, Potassium: 195 mg, Phosphorus: 20 mg	1 medium apple	5 minutes
Blueberries	Fresh blueberries	Wash and pat dry.	Calories: 84, Potassiu	1 cup	5 minutes

		Can be added to yogurt or eaten as a snack.	m: 114 mg, Phosphorus: 18 mg		
Grapes	Fresh grapes	Wash thoroughly. Eat raw or freeze for a cool treat.	Calories: 69, Potassium: 191 mg, Phosphorus: 20 mg	1 cup	5 minutes
Pineapples	Fresh pineapple	Peel and core. Slice into chunks. Can be eaten fresh or grilled.	Calories: 82, Potassium: 180 mg, Phosphorus: 13 mg	1 cup	10 minutes

Strawb erries	Fresh strawbe rries	Wash and hull. Eat raw or add to salads and desserts.	Calories : 49, Potassiu m: 153 mg, Phosph orus: 17 mg	1 cup	5 minutes
Pears	Fresh pears	Wash and core. Slice or eat whole. Can be eaten raw or poache d.	Calories : 102, Potassiu m: 206 mg, Phosph orus: 12 mg	1 mediu m pear	5 minutes
Peache s	Fresh peaches	Wash, peel, and slice. Eat raw	Calories : 59, Potassiu m: 285 mg,	1 mediu m peach	10 minutes

		or use in baking.	Phosph orus: 13 mg		
Cherri es	Fresh cherries	Wash and remove pits. Eat raw or use in desserts.	Calories : 63, Potassiu m: 222 mg, Phosph orus: 18 mg	1 cup	5 minutes
Melons	Cantalo upe or honeyd ew	Wash, peel, and cut into chunks. Eat fresh or add to salads.	Calories : 60 (cantalo upe), Potassiu m: 267 mg, Phosph orus: 19 mg	1 cup	10 minutes
Plums	Fresh plums	Wash and slice.	Calories : 30, Potassiu m	1 mediu m plum	5 minutes

		Eat raw or use in jams and preserves.	m: 104 mg, Phosphorus: 16 mg		
Kiwi	Fresh kiwi	Peel and slice. Eat raw or add to smoothies.	Calories: 42, Potassium: 215 mg, Phosphorus: 34 mg	1 medium kiwi	5 minutes
Raspberries	Fresh raspberries	Wash and pat dry. Eat raw or add to yogurt and salads.	Calories: 65, Potassium: 186 mg, Phosphorus: 32 mg	1 cup	5 minutes

Blackberries	Fresh blackberries	Wash and pat dry. Eat raw or add to smoothies and cereals.	Calories: 43, Potassium: 233 mg, Phosphorus: 22 mg	1 cup	5 minutes
Pomegranates	Fresh pomegranate	Peel and remove seeds. Eat seeds raw or add to salads.	Calories: 83, Potassium: 205 mg, Phosphorus: 36 mg	1/2 cup seeds	10 minutes
Apricots	Fresh apricots	Wash and slice. Eat raw or use in baking.	Calories: 17, Potassium: 91 mg, Phosphorus: 12 mg	2 medium apricots	5 minutes

This table provides an overview of some kidney-friendly fruits, highlighting their nutritional content and how they can be prepared and served. Each fruit is selected for its relatively low levels of potassium and phosphorus, making them suitable for those managing kidney disease.

Grains and Starches

Here's a detailed table covering grains and starches that are suitable for a kidney-friendly diet, including ingredients, instructions, nutritional information, serving size, and cooking time:

Ingredient	Instructions	Nutritional Information (Per Serving)	Serving Size	Cooking Time
White Rice	Rinse before cooking. Cook in a rice cooker or on the stovetop with a 1:2 rice-to-water ratio.	Calories: 205, Carbs: 45g, Protein: 4g, Fat: 0g	1 cup cooked	15-20 minutes
Pearl Barley	Rinse before	Calories: 200,	1 cup cooked	30-40 minutes

	cooking. Boil in water for 30-40 minutes until tender.	Carbs: 44g, Protein: 4g, Fat: 1g		
Couscous	Cook with a 1:1.5 couscous-to-water ratio. Steam or simmer for 5 minutes until fluffy.	Calories: 176, Carbs: 36g, Protein: 6g, Fat: 0g	1 cup cooked	5 minutes
Quinoa	Rinse before cooking. Use a 1:2 quinoa-to-water	Calories: 222, Carbs: 39g, Protein: 8g, Fat: 4g	1 cup cooked	15 minutes

	ratio. Simmer for 15 minutes.			
White Cornmeal	Cook in boiling water, stirring frequently for about 20 minutes until thickened.	Calories: 120, Carbs: 30g, Protein: 3g, Fat: 0g	1/2 cup cooked	20 minutes
Polenta	Cook in water or broth, stirring frequently until thickened (about 30 minutes).	Calories: 140, Carbs: 30g, Protein: 3g, Fat: 1g	1/2 cup cooked	30 minutes

Bulgur Wheat	Rinse before cooking. Boil in water for 12-15 minutes or soak in hot water until tender.	Calories: 151, Carbs: 33g, Protein: 5g, Fat: 0g	1 cup cooked	12-15 minutes
Farro	Rinse before cooking. Boil in water for 30-40 minutes until tender.	Calories: 220, Carbs: 45g, Protein: 7g, Fat: 1g	1 cup cooked	30-40 minutes
Amaranth	Rinse before cooking. Use a 1:2 amaranth-	Calories: 251, Carbs: 46g,	1 cup cooked	20 minutes

	to-water ratio. Simmer for 20 minutes.	Protein: 9g, Fat: 4g		
Oats	Cook with a 1:2 oats-to-water ratio. Simmer for 5-10 minutes.	Calories: 154, Carbs: 27g, Protein: 6g, Fat: 3g	1 cup cooked	5-10 minutes
Brown Rice	Rinse before cooking. Use a 1:2 brown rice-to-water ratio. Simmer for 45 minutes.	Calories: 215, Carbs: 45g, Protein: 5g, Fat: 1.5g	1 cup cooked	45 minutes
Wild Rice	Rinse before	Calories: 166,	1 cup cooked	45-60 minutes

	cooking. Boil in water for 45-60 minutes until tender.	Carbs: 35g, Protein: 7g, Fat: 0.5g		
Rye	Cook in water or broth, simmer for about 30 minutes until tender.	Calories: 115, Carbs: 24g, Protein: 3g, Fat: 0.5g	1/2 cup cooked	30 minutes
Buckwheat	Rinse before cooking. Use a 1:2 buckwheat-to-water ratio. Simmer	Calories: 155, Carbs: 33g, Protein: 6g, Fat: 1g	1 cup cooked	10-15 minutes

	for 10-15 minutes.			
Spelt	Rinse before cooking. Boil in water for 30 minutes or until tender.	Calories: 198, Carbs: 41g, Protein: 7g, Fat: 1g	1 cup cooked	30 minutes

This table provides a comprehensive overview of various grains and starches suitable for a kidney-friendly diet. It includes instructions for preparation, nutritional information per serving, typical serving sizes, and approximate cooking times. This information helps guide individuals in making informed dietary choices that align with managing kidney disease effectively.

Proteins

Here is a detailed table for the "Proteins" section in relation to "The Essential Foods Lists For Kidney Disease":

Protein Ingredient	Instruction	Nutritional Information (per serving)	Serving Size	Cooking Time
Chicken Breast	Grill or bake with minimal seasoning. Avoid skin.	165 calories, 31g protein, 0g carbs, 3.6g fat	3 oz	20-25 minutes
Egg Whites	Scramble or cook as an omelet. Avoid adding cheese.	17 calories, 3.6g protein, 0g carbs, 0.1g fat	3 large egg whites	5-7 minutes
Tilapia	Bake or grill with	110 calories,	3 oz	15-20 minutes

	a squeeze of lemon and herbs.	23g protein, 0g carbs, 1.5g fat		
Turkey Breast	Roast or grill with light seasoning.	135 calories, 30g protein, 0g carbs, 1g fat	3 oz	25-30 minutes
Cod	Bake with olive oil and fresh herbs.	90 calories, 20g protein, 0g carbs, 0.7g fat	3 oz	15-20 minutes
Tofu	Stir-fry or bake with vegetables.	70 calories, 8g protein, 2g carbs, 4g fat	3 oz	10-15 minutes

Lentils	Boil until tender. Can be used in soups or salads.	230 calories, 18g protein, 40g carbs, 0.8g fat	1 cup cooked	20-25 minutes
Pork Loin	Roast with minimal seasoning.	143 calories, 26g protein, 0g carbs, 4g fat	3 oz	25-30 minutes
Greek Yogurt (plain, non-fat)	Eat plain or add low-potassium fruits.	100 calories, 10g protein, 6g carbs, 0g fat	1 cup	0 minutes (ready-to-eat)
Cottage Cheese (low-sodium)	Eat as is or add to salads.	206 calories, 28g protein, 6g carbs, 9g fat	1 cup	0 minutes (ready-to-eat)

Shrimp	Boil or grill with herbs and spices.	84 calories, 18g protein, 1g carbs, 1g fat	3 oz	5-7 minutes
Salmon	Bake or grill with lemon and herbs.	206 calories, 22g protein, 0g carbs, 13g fat	3 oz	15-20 minutes
Chicken Thigh (skinless)	Bake or grill with minimal seasoning.	209 calories, 26g protein, 0g carbs, 11g fat	3 oz	20-25 minutes
Venison	Roast or grill with light seasoning.	158 calories, 30g protein, 0g carbs, 2g fat	3 oz	25-30 minutes

Whitefish	Bake or grill with herbs.	130 calories, 26g protein, 0g carbs, 2g fat	3 oz	15-20 minutes

This table provides a comprehensive overview of kidney-friendly protein sources, including instructions for preparation, nutritional information per serving, typical serving sizes, and estimated cooking times.

Dairy and Alternatives

Here is a comprehensive table about dairy and alternatives suitable for managing kidney disease:

Ingredient	Instruction	Nutritional Information (per serving)	Serving Size	Cooking Time
Almond Milk (unsweetened)	Shake well before use. Use in place of regular milk for drinking or in recipes.	Calories: 30, Protein: 1g, Fat: 2.5g, Carbohydrates: 1g, Potassium: 160mg	1 cup	N/A
Rice Milk (unenriched)	Shake well before use. Ideal for cereal or as a milk	Calories: 50, Protein: 1g, Fat: 1g, Carbohyd	1 cup	N/A

	substitute in recipes.	rates: 10g, Potassium : 200mg		
Coconut Milk (unsweetened)	Shake before use. Use in smoothies, curries, or as a milk replacement.	Calories: 45, Protein: 0g, Fat: 4.5g, Carbohydrates: 1g, Potassium : 60mg	1 cup	N/A
Soy Milk (unsweetened)	Shake well before use. Use as a dairy alternative for drinking or cooking.	Calories: 80, Protein: 7g, Fat: 4g, Carbohydrates: 4g, Potassium : 300mg	1 cup	N/A

Low-Fat Cottage Cheese	Use as a topping or snack. Mix with fruits or vegetables for added flavor.	Calories: 90, Protein: 11g, Fat: 2g, Carbohydrates: 4g, Potassium: 200mg	1/2 cup	N/A
Ricotta Cheese (part-skim)	Use in recipes like lasagna or as a filling for pasta.	Calories: 300, Protein: 14g, Fat: 16g, Carbohydrates: 11g, Potassium: 250mg	1/2 cup	N/A
Greek Yogurt (plain, low-fat)	Use as a snack or in smoothies. Can also be used in cooking as	Calories: 100, Protein: 10g, Fat: 0g, Carbohydrates: 6g,	1 cup	N/A

	a substitute for sour cream.	Potassium: 150mg		
Kefir (low-fat)	Drink straight or use in smoothies. Fermented milk with probiotic benefits.	Calories: 100, Protein: 6g, Fat: 2g, Carbohydrates: 12g, Potassium: 200mg	1 cup	N/A
Goat Cheese (soft, low-fat)	Use as a topping for salads or as a spread.	Calories: 75, Protein: 5g, Fat: 6g, Carbohydrates: 0g, Potassium: 125mg	1 ounce	N/A

Skim Milk	Use for drinking or in cooking. Lower in fat compared to whole milk.	Calories: 80, Protein: 8g, Fat: 0g, Carbohydrates: 12g, Potassium: 400mg	1 cup	N/A
Low-Fat Plain Yogurt	Use as a snack, in smoothies, or as a cooking ingredient.	Calories: 100, Protein: 6g, Fat: 2g, Carbohydrates: 15g, Potassium: 250mg	1 cup	N/A
Almond-Based Creamer	Use in coffee or tea as a dairy-free alternative.	Calories: 15, Protein: 0g, Fat: 1g, Carbohydrates: 1g,	1 tablespoon	N/A

		Potassium: 40mg		
Oat Milk	Shake before use. Suitable for drinking or cooking.	Calories: 120, Protein: 3g, Fat: 5g, Carbohydrates: 16g, Potassium: 350mg	1 cup	N/A
Pea Protein Milk	Shake well before use. Ideal for those with nut allergies.	Calories: 70, Protein: 8g, Fat: 4g, Carbohydrates: 1g, Potassium: 330mg	1 cup	N/A
Cashew Milk	Shake before use. Use as a milk	Calories: 25, Protein: 1g, Fat:	1 cup	N/A

	substitute in various recipes.	2g, Carbohyd rates: 1g, Potassium : 60mg		

This table provides a detailed overview of dairy and dairy alternatives suitable for individuals managing kidney disease, including instructions for use, nutritional information, serving sizes, and cooking times where applicable.

Beverages

Here is a comprehensive table on beverages that are suitable for kidney disease, including ingredients, instructions, nutritional information, serving size, and cooking time.

Beverage	Ingredients	Instructions	Nutritional Information	Serving Size	Preparation Time
Cucumber Mint Water	1 cucumber, sliced 10 fresh mint leaves 1 liter water	Combine cucumber slices and mint leaves in a pitcher. Add water and refrigerate for	Calories: 10 Potassium: 10 mg Sodium: 0 mg Phosphorus: 0 mg	1 cup	5 minutes

		at least 1 hour before serving.			
Lemonade (Low Potassium)	1 lemon, juiced 2 cups water 1 tablespoon honey (optional)	Mix lemon juice, water, and honey (if using) in a pitcher. Stir well and serve chilled.	Calories: 50 Potassium: 20 mg Sodium: 0 mg Phosphorus: 0 mg	1 cup	10 minutes
Apple Cinnamon Tea	1 apple, sliced 1 cinnamon stick 2	Steep apple slices and cinnamon stick in	Calories: 30 Potassium: 120 mg Sodium	1 cup	10 minutes

	cups boiling water	boiling water for 5-10 minutes. Strain and serve.	m: 0 mg Phosphorus: 0 mg		
Herbal Chamomile Tea	1 chamomile tea bag 1 cup boiling water	Steep tea bag in boiling water for 5 minutes. Remove tea bag and serve.	Calories: 0 Potassium: 5 mg Sodium: 0 mg Phosphorus: 0 mg	1 cup	5 minutes
Berry Infused Water	1/2 cup strawberries, sliced 1/2 cup	Combine berries in a pitcher with	Calories: 15 Potassium: 15 mg 	1 cup	5 minutes

	raspber ries 1 liter water	water. Refrige rate for at least 1 hour before serving.	>Sodiu m: 0 mg >Phosp horus: 0 mg		
Green Tea (Decaff einated)	1 decaffei nated green tea bag 1 cup boiling water	Steep tea bag in boiling water for 3-5 minutes . Remov e tea bag and serve.	Calories : 0 P otassiu m: 20 mg >Sodiu m: 0 mg >Phosp horus: 0 mg	1 cup	5 minutes
Peach Iced Tea	1 cup brewed tea (cooled) 1/ 2 cup	Combi ne cooled tea and peach slices in	Calories : 60 Potassiu m: 70 mg 	1 cup	15 minutes

	peach slices 1 tablespoon honey (optional)	a pitcher. Add honey if desired. Refrigerate for 1 hour before serving.	>Sodium: 0 mg Phosphorus: 5 mg		
Watermelon Juice	2 cups watermelon chunks 1 tablespoon lime juice	Blend watermelon chunks until smooth. Strain if desired. Stir in lime juice and serve chilled.	Calories: 50 Potassium: 150 mg Sodium: 0 mg Phosphorus: 10 mg	1 cup	10 minutes

| **Ginger Lemon Tea** | 1 tablespoon fresh ginger, sliced
1 lemon, juiced
2 cups boiling water | Steep ginger in boiling water for 5 minutes. Add lemon juice and stir. Serve hot or chilled. | Calories: 15
Potassium: 50 mg
Sodium: 0 mg
Phosphorus: 5 mg | 1 cup | 10 minutes |
| **Coconut Water** | 1 cup 100% coconut water | Pour coconut water into a glass and serve chilled. | Calories: 45
Potassium: 600 mg
Sodium: 60 mg
Phosp | 1 cup | 0 minutes |

			horus: 40 mg		
Herbal Pepper mint Tea	1 pepper mint tea bag 1 cup boiling water	Steep tea bag in boiling water for 5 minutes. Remove tea bag and serve.	Calories: 0 Potassium: 5 mg Sodium: 0 mg Phosphorus: 0 mg	1 cup	5 minutes
Orange Infused Water	1 orange, sliced 1 liter water	Combine orange slices in a pitcher with water. Refrigerate for at least	Calories: 20 Potassium: 30 mg Sodium: 0 mg Phosp	1 cup	5 minutes

		1 hour before serving.	horus: 0 mg		
Strawberry Mint Lemonade	1/2 cup strawberries, sliced 1 lemon, juiced 2 cups water 10 mint leaves	Blend strawberries and lemon juice. Mix with water and add mint leaves. Serve chilled.	Calories: 40 Potassium: 25 mg Sodium: 0 mg Phosphorus: 0 mg	1 cup	15 minutes
Pineapple Cucumber Water	1/2 cup pineapple chunks 1/2 cucumber,	Combine pineapple chunks and cucumber	Calories: 20 Potassium: 30 mg Sodium: 0	1 cup	5 minutes

	sliced 1 liter water	slices in a pitcher. Add water and refriger ate for at least 1 hour before serving.	mg Phosp horus: 0 mg		
Apple Ginger Sparkle r	1 cup apple juice (unswee tened) 1/2 teaspoo n fresh ginger, grated 1 cup	Mix apple juice and ginger. Top with sparklin g water and serve chilled.	Calories : 80 Potassiu m: 120 mg Sodiu m: 0 mg Phosp horus: 10 mg	1 cup	5 minutes

	sparklin g water				

This table offers a range of beverages that are suitable for those managing kidney disease, providing options that are both refreshing and aligned with dietary needs.

Chapter 2: Foods to Avoid for Kidney Disease

High-Potassium Foods

Here is a detailed table outlining high-potassium foods to avoid for managing kidney disease, along with explanations of why they should be limited or avoided.

Food	Why to Avoid
Bananas	Bananas are high in potassium, which can be harmful to individuals with kidney disease as it may cause hyperkalemia (elevated potassium levels) that can affect heart function.
Oranges	Oranges and orange juice are rich in potassium. Excess potassium can strain the kidneys, worsening the disease and causing imbalances in electrolytes.

Potatoes	Potatoes contain significant amounts of potassium. Consuming them in large quantities can lead to dangerous increases in potassium levels, which the kidneys may not filter effectively.
Sweet Potatoes	Sweet potatoes are also high in potassium. Like regular potatoes, they can contribute to elevated potassium levels, exacerbating kidney-related health issues.
Tomatoes	Tomatoes, including tomato sauce and paste, are high in potassium. Overconsumption can lead to potassium buildup, stressing the kidneys and increasing health risks.
Spinach	Spinach is very high in potassium. It can be particularly problematic for kidney patients as it may lead

	to excessive potassium levels in the bloodstream.
Avocados	Avocados have high potassium content. Excessive intake can overwhelm the kidneys' ability to regulate potassium levels, posing a risk to those with kidney disease.
Dried Fruits	Dried fruits, such as raisins and apricots, have concentrated levels of potassium. They can contribute to high potassium levels quickly, complicating kidney management.
Beets	Beets are rich in potassium. Regular consumption can lead to elevated potassium levels, which can be problematic for individuals with compromised kidney function.

Melons	Melons, including cantaloupe and honeydew, are high in potassium. Excessive consumption can result in potassium overload, stressing the kidneys and impacting overall health.
Chili Peppers	Chili peppers contain high amounts of potassium. For those with kidney disease, excessive potassium intake can disrupt electrolyte balance and kidney function.
Bran Cereals	Bran cereals are high in potassium. Consuming them frequently can lead to increased potassium levels in the blood, which may be harmful to individuals with kidney issues.
Nuts and Seeds	Many nuts and seeds are high in potassium. Regular consumption can lead to elevated potassium levels,

	which may contribute to worsening kidney disease symptoms.
Coconut Water	Coconut water is known for its high potassium content. Regular intake can cause potassium buildup, which is risky for people with impaired kidney function.
Fish (Certain Types)	Some types of fish, like salmon and tuna, are high in potassium. Excessive intake of these can lead to increased potassium levels, putting additional strain on the kidneys.

This table highlights high-potassium foods that should be avoided by individuals managing kidney disease. Limiting or avoiding these foods helps prevent complications related to potassium imbalances and supports better kidney health.

High-Phosphorus Foods

high-phosphorus foods and why they should be avoided for individuals with kidney disease, as outlined in "The Essential Foods Lists For Kidney Disease":

High-Phosphorus Food	Reason to Avoid	Phosphorus Content (per serving)	Alternative Options
Dairy Products	Dairy products are rich in phosphorus, which can accumulate in the blood if the kidneys are not functioning properly. High phosphorus levels can lead to bone and	1 cup milk: 250 mg 1 oz cheddar cheese: 175 mg	Almond milk (unenriched) Rice milk (unenriched)

	heart problems.		
Nuts and Seeds	Nuts and seeds contain high levels of phosphorus, which can be difficult for compromised kidneys to process. Excess phosphorus can contribute to calcium and bone issues.	1 oz almonds: 140 mg 1 oz sunflower seeds: 190 mg	Fresh fruits Vegetables
Meat and Poultry (processed)	Processed meats often contain added phosphorus as preservatives or flavor	2 oz processed ham: 300 mg 2 oz bacon: 200 mg	Fresh, unprocessed meats Tofu

	enhancers. High phosphorus levels can affect bone health and cardiovascular function.		
Fish (certain types)	Some types of fish, especially processed or canned, are high in phosphorus. Excess phosphorus from these sources can be harmful to kidney function.	3 oz canned tuna: 250 mg 3 oz salmon: 300 mg	Fresh fish Chicken breast
Whole Grains	Whole grains are high in phosphorus	1 cup cooked quinoa: 280 mg 1	White rice Refined pasta

	due to their bran content. While they offer many nutrients, their phosphorus content can be excessive for individuals with kidney disease.	cup whole wheat pasta: 250 mg	
Chocolate and Cocoa	Chocolate and cocoa are high in phosphorus, which can contribute to imbalances in those with kidney disease. They can also be high in	1 oz dark chocolate: 150 mg 1 cup cocoa powder: 700 mg	Fruit-based desserts Low-phosphorus snacks

	potassium and sodium.		
Beer and Soft Drinks	Many beers and soft drinks contain added phosphates for flavor and preservation. Consuming these beverages can increase phosphorus levels in the blood.	12 oz beer: 150 mg 12 oz cola: 100 mg	Herbal teas Fruit-infused waters
Fast Foods	Fast foods often contain high levels of phosphorus from additives and preservatives used to	1 burger: 250 mg 1 serving fries: 200 mg	Homemade, low-phosphorus meals Salads

	enhance flavor and shelf life. This can contribute to higher phosphorus levels.		
Packaged Snacks	Packaged snacks often have added phosphates for preservation and flavor. Regular consumption can lead to excessive phosphorus intake.	1 oz potato chips: 150 mg 1 oz pretzels: 200 mg	Fresh fruit Vegetable sticks
Processed Cheese	Processed cheese contains added	1 slice processed cheese: 150 mg 1 oz	Low-phosphorus cheese options Fresh cheese

	phosphorus and preservatives that can increase phosphorus levels in the blood.	cheese spread: 250 mg	
Legumes	Many legumes are high in phosphorus, which can be difficult to manage in the diet of someone with kidney disease. Excess phosphorus can impact kidney and bone health.	1 cup cooked lentils: 365 mg 1 cup cooked chickpeas: 250 mg	Low-phosphorus vegetables Lean meats

This table highlights the key high-phosphorus foods to avoid and explains why managing phosphorus intake is crucial for individuals with kidney disease. It also provides alternative options to help maintain a balanced diet while managing phosphorus levels effectively.

High-Sodium Foods

Here's a detailed table about high-sodium foods and why they should be avoided for kidney disease management:

High-Sodium Food	Why You Should Avoid It
Canned Soups	Often contain high levels of sodium used as a preservative, which can contribute to fluid retention and increased blood pressure, exacerbating kidney issues.
Frozen Meals	Pre-packaged frozen meals frequently have high sodium content to enhance flavor and shelf life, which can stress the kidneys and contribute to high blood pressure.
Processed Meats	Items like bacon, ham, and sausage are cured or preserved with large amounts of sodium, which can lead to fluid retention and further strain on the kidneys.

Salted Snacks	Chips, pretzels, and salted nuts are high in sodium, which can contribute to elevated blood pressure and make it harder for kidneys to manage fluid balance.
Pickles and Olives	These foods are preserved in brine, which contains high amounts of sodium, increasing sodium intake and contributing to kidney stress and high blood pressure.
Soy Sauce	Contains very high sodium levels used for flavoring; excessive sodium can worsen kidney function and elevate blood pressure.
Instant Noodles	Often high in sodium due to flavoring packets, which can contribute to hypertension and kidney strain.
Canned Vegetables	Like canned soups, they often include added sodium for

	preservation, which can negatively impact kidney function and increase blood pressure.
Cheese	Many cheeses are high in sodium, which can exacerbate fluid retention and increase strain on the kidneys.
Fast Food	Typically high in sodium due to added salts and preservatives, contributing to poor kidney health and elevated blood pressure.
Prepared Sauces	Sauces like barbecue, teriyaki, and pasta sauces often contain high amounts of sodium to enhance flavor, which can worsen kidney function.
Salty Condiments	Items like ketchup, mustard, and salad dressings often contain added sodium, which can contribute to high blood pressure and kidney stress.

Meat Jerky	Contains high levels of sodium used for curing and flavoring, which can exacerbate kidney disease and hypertension.
Commercially Baked Goods	Items like cookies, cakes, and pastries often have high sodium content to enhance taste and preserve freshness, which can be harmful to kidney health.
Pre-packaged Seasonings	Many seasoning blends and salt substitutes contain added sodium, which can increase overall sodium intake and negatively impact kidney function.

High-sodium foods can significantly impact individuals with kidney disease by increasing fluid retention, raising blood pressure, and putting additional stress on the kidneys. Sodium is a key factor in regulating fluid balance in the body, and excessive intake can lead to complications such as edema and hypertension. Avoiding these foods helps manage kidney health, control blood pressure, and prevent the progression of kidney disease.

High-Oxalate Foods

Here's a detailed table about high-oxalate foods and why they should be avoided for kidney disease:

High-Oxalate Food	Why You Should Avoid It
Spinach	Spinach is very high in oxalates, which can contribute to the formation of kidney stones. Consuming large amounts can exacerbate kidney problems, particularly in individuals with a history of stone formation.
Rhubarb	Rhubarb has a high oxalate content that can increase the risk of developing kidney stones. It is best to avoid it to minimize the risk of kidney complications.
Beets	Beets contain significant amounts of oxalates, which can contribute to the formation of kidney stones.

	Limiting beet consumption helps manage oxalate levels and supports kidney health.
Nuts	Various nuts, including almonds and cashews, are high in oxalates. Regular consumption can increase the risk of kidney stones and exacerbate kidney disease symptoms.
Chocolate	Chocolate, particularly dark chocolate, is rich in oxalates. Frequent consumption can contribute to elevated oxalate levels, which can be harmful for individuals with kidney disease.
Tea (Black and Green)	Both black and green teas are high in oxalates, which can contribute to kidney stone formation. Limiting tea consumption can help manage oxalate levels and reduce kidney strain.

Sweet Potatoes	Sweet potatoes contain moderate levels of oxalates, which can contribute to kidney stone formation. Reducing their intake helps control oxalate levels and supports kidney health.
Soy Products	Soybeans and soy-based products are high in oxalates. Regular consumption can elevate oxalate levels in the body, increasing the risk of kidney stones and exacerbating kidney issues.
Swiss Chard	Swiss chard is very high in oxalates and can contribute to kidney stone formation. Avoiding it helps manage oxalate levels and supports kidney function.
Okra	Okra contains high amounts of oxalates, which can contribute to kidney stone formation. Limiting its

	consumption helps prevent the potential complications associated with high oxalate levels.
Fennel	Fennel has a moderate amount of oxalates. Regular consumption can contribute to elevated oxalate levels, which may impact kidney health negatively.
Parsnips	Parsnips contain significant oxalates, which can contribute to kidney stone formation. Managing intake helps control oxalate levels and support kidney function.
Amaranth	Amaranth is high in oxalates and can increase the risk of kidney stones. Limiting its consumption helps manage oxalate levels and reduce the risk of kidney complications.

Buckwheat	Buckwheat contains oxalates that can contribute to the formation of kidney stones. Reducing its intake helps maintain lower oxalate levels and supports kidney health.
Celery	Celery contains moderate levels of oxalates. Regular consumption can contribute to elevated oxalate levels, which may impact kidney health negatively.

High-oxalate foods can contribute to the formation of kidney stones, which can further exacerbate kidney disease. Managing oxalate intake is crucial for individuals with kidney issues to help prevent complications and support overall kidney function. Avoiding or limiting these high-oxalate foods can help maintain lower oxalate levels in the body and reduce the risk of kidney-related problems.

Sugary Foods and Drinks

Here is a detailed table on sugary foods and drinks to avoid for kidney disease, explaining why they should be avoided:

Sugary Food/Drink	Why to Avoid	Nutritional Information (per serving)
Regular Soda	High in added sugars and calories, which can lead to weight gain and worsen kidney disease. Excess sugar can also increase blood pressure and contribute to diabetes, which is detrimental to kidney health.	Calories: 150 Sugars: 39 g Potassium: 0 mg Sodium: 40 mg
Fruit Juices (e.g., Orange Juice, Apple Juice)	Often high in natural sugars and calories, with minimal fiber	Calories: 110 (8 oz) Sugars: 25 g Potassium: 330

	compared to whole fruits. Can lead to spikes in blood sugar and contribute to kidney stress.	mg Sodium: 2 mg
Energy Drinks	Contain high levels of sugars and caffeine. Excessive sugar intake can increase the risk of diabetes and high blood pressure, which negatively impacts kidney function.	Calories: 160 Sugars: 42 g Potassium: 200 mg Sodium: 200 mg
Sweetened Coffee Drinks (e.g., Flavored Lattes, Coffee with Syrups)	High in sugars and often high in caffeine, which can strain the kidneys and increase blood pressure. Sugary syrups contribute to excessive calorie intake.	Calories: 200 (medium) Sugars: 30 g Potassium: 300 mg Sodium: 100 mg

Candy Bars	High in added sugars and fats, contributing to weight gain and increased risk of diabetes. Excess sugar can exacerbate kidney issues and worsen overall health.	Calories: 250 Sugars: 30 g Potassium: 100 mg Sodium: 150 mg
Baked Goods (e.g., Muffins, Cookies, Donuts)	Often high in sugars, fats, and calories, leading to weight gain and higher risk of diabetes. These can negatively affect kidney health and increase blood pressure.	Calories: 300 (muffin) Suga rs: 40 g Potassium: 200 mg Sodium: 200 mg
Sugary Cereals	High in added sugars and low in nutritional value. Excessive sugar intake can	Calories: 150 (1 cup) Sugars: 15 g Potassium: 250

	contribute to weight gain and worsen kidney disease. Fiber content is often insufficient.	mg Sodium: 200 mg
Sweetened Yogurts	Often contain high amounts of added sugars, which can lead to increased calorie intake and spikes in blood sugar. This can exacerbate kidney problems and increase cardiovascular risk.	Calories: 150 (6 oz) Sugars: 20 g Potassium: 250 mg Sodium: 70 mg
Ice Cream	High in sugars and fats, contributing to excessive calorie intake and potential weight gain. This can strain the kidneys	Calories: 200 (1/2 cup) Sugars: 20 g Potassium: 150 mg Sodium: 60 mg

	and worsen kidney disease.	
Packaged Fruit Snacks	High in added sugars and often low in nutritional value. Excessive sugar intake can lead to weight gain and negatively affect kidney function.	Calories: 100 (1 serving) Sugars: 20 g Potassium: 50 mg Sodium: 15 mg
Granola Bars (sweetened)	Frequently high in sugars and may contain unhealthy fats. Excessive sugar can increase the risk of diabetes and high blood pressure, impacting kidney health.	Calories: 200 (1 bar) Sugars: 18 g Potassium: 150 mg Sodium: 100 mg
Soft Drinks (Diet)	While lower in calories, diet sodas often contain	Calories: 0 Sugars: 0 g Potassium:

	artificial sweeteners which may not be ideal for kidney health. They can also encourage a preference for sweet flavors.	0 mg Sodium: 40 mg
Sweetened Tea	High in sugars and calories. Excessive sugar intake can contribute to weight gain and increase the risk of diabetes, which affects kidney health.	Calories: 80 (12 oz) Sugars: 20 g Potassium: 150 mg Sodium: 10 mg
Flavored Milk (e.g., Chocolate Milk)	Contains added sugars and calories, which can contribute to weight gain and worsen kidney disease. Regular consumption can	Calories: 190 (8 oz) Sugars: 26 g Potassium: 350 mg Sodium: 110 mg

	impact kidney function.	

This table outlines various sugary foods and drinks to avoid for managing kidney disease, explaining how high sugar content can exacerbate health issues related to kidney function. Avoiding these items helps in maintaining a balanced diet and managing kidney health effectively.

Alcohol and Caffeine

Here's a detailed table on alcohol and caffeine, outlining why they should be avoided for individuals with kidney disease:

Substance	Why to Avoid	Effects on Kidney Disease	Examples
Alcohol	Alcohol can increase blood pressure and contribute to dehydration, both of which can exacerbate kidney disease. Excessive alcohol intake can lead to liver damage, further	- Raises blood pressure, putting additional strain on the kidneys. - Increases risk of dehydration, which can affect kidney function. - Interferes with the effectiveness of	- Beer - Wine - Liquor - Cocktails - Liqueurs

	complicating kidney function. Additionally, alcohol can interfere with the metabolism of medications commonly prescribed for kidney disease. It may also contribute to the development of chronic diseases such as diabetes, which can further impair kidney function.	medications for kidney disease. - Contributes to liver damage, impacting overall health and kidney function.	

| **Caffeine** | Caffeine can act as a diuretic, leading to increased urine production and potential dehydration. For individuals with kidney disease, managing fluid balance is crucial, and excessive caffeine can disrupt this balance. Additionally, caffeine may increase blood pressure and contribute to | - Acts as a diuretic, which can lead to dehydration and electrolyte imbalances.
- Can increase blood pressure, adding extra strain on the kidneys.
- May contribute to the progression of kidney disease if consumed in excess. | - Coffee
- Black tea
- Energy drinks
- Cola
- Green tea |

	worsening kidney function over time.		

This table provides a clear overview of why alcohol and caffeine should be avoided for individuals with kidney disease. It highlights their potential negative effects on kidney function and overall health, helping guide dietary choices for better management of the condition.

Chapter 3: Recipes and Meal Ideas

Breakfast Ideas

Low-Potassium Smoothie

- **Ingredients:** 1 cup blueberries, 1/2 banana, 1 cup almond milk (unenriched), 1 tablespoon chia seeds
- **Instructions:** Blend all ingredients until smooth. Pour into a glass and serve immediately.
- **Nutritional Information:** Calories: 190, Potassium: 200 mg, Sodium: 30 mg, Phosphorus: 80 mg
- **Serving Size:** 1 cup
- **Cooking Time:** 5 minutes

Kidney-Friendly Omelet

- **Ingredients:** 2 egg whites, 1/4 cup bell peppers (chopped), 1/4 cup spinach (cooked), 1/4 cup mushrooms (sliced), 1 teaspoon olive oil
- **Instructions:** Heat olive oil in a non-stick pan. Add vegetables and sauté for 2-3 minutes. Pour egg whites over the vegetables and cook until set. Fold omelet and serve.

- **Nutritional Information:** Calories: 120, Potassium: 150 mg, Sodium: 40 mg, Phosphorus: 60 mg
- **Serving Size:** 1 omelet
- **Cooking Time:** 10 minutes

Lunch Ideas

Salad with Low-Potassium Veggies

- **Ingredients:** 2 cups mixed greens, 1/2 cup cherry tomatoes, 1/4 cup cucumber (sliced), 1/4 cup shredded carrots, 1 tablespoon olive oil, 1 tablespoon balsamic vinegar
- **Instructions:** Toss mixed greens, tomatoes, cucumber, and carrots in a bowl. Drizzle with olive oil and balsamic vinegar before serving.
- **Nutritional Information:** Calories: 150, Potassium: 300 mg, Sodium: 30 mg, Phosphorus: 40 mg
- **Serving Size:** 1 bowl
- **Cooking Time:** 10 minutes

Turkey and Veggie Wrap

- **Ingredients:** 1 whole wheat tortilla, 3 slices turkey breast, 1/4 avocado (sliced), 1/4 cup shredded lettuce, 1 tablespoon low-sodium mayonnaise

- **Instructions:** Spread mayonnaise on the tortilla. Layer with turkey, avocado, and lettuce. Roll up and slice in half.
- **Nutritional Information:** Calories: 250, Potassium: 350 mg, Sodium: 200 mg, Phosphorus: 90 mg
- **Serving Size:** 1 wrap
- **Cooking Time:** 10 minutes

Dinner Ideas

Grilled Chicken with Steamed Veggies

- **Ingredients:** 1 boneless, skinless chicken breast, 1 cup broccoli florets, 1 cup cauliflower florets, 1 tablespoon olive oil, salt and pepper to taste
- **Instructions:** Season chicken with salt and pepper. Grill over medium heat for 6-7 minutes per side or until cooked through. Steam broccoli and cauliflower until tender. Drizzle olive oil over vegetables.
- **Nutritional Information:** Calories: 300, Potassium: 600 mg, Sodium: 100 mg, Phosphorus: 120 mg
- **Serving Size:** 1 chicken breast with 1 cup vegetables
- **Cooking Time:** 20 minutes

Fish Tacos with Cabbage Slaw

- **Ingredients:** 1 fish fillet (such as tilapia), 2 small tortillas, 1 cup shredded cabbage, 1/4 cup shredded carrots, 2 tablespoons lime juice, 1 tablespoon olive oil
- **Instructions:** Grill or bake fish fillet until cooked through. Mix cabbage, carrots, lime juice, and olive oil to make slaw. Serve fish in tortillas topped with cabbage slaw.
- **Nutritional Information:** Calories: 250, Potassium: 400 mg, Sodium: 150 mg, Phosphorus: 100 mg
- **Serving Size:** 2 tacos
- **Cooking Time:** 15 minutes

Snacks and Appetizers

Fresh Fruit Slices

- **Ingredients:** 1 apple, 1/2 cup blueberries, 1 pear
- **Instructions:** Slice apple and pear. Serve with blueberries on the side.
- **Nutritional Information:** Calories: 100, Potassium: 200 mg, Sodium: 1 mg, Phosphorus: 30 mg
- **Serving Size:** 1 serving (1 apple, 1/2 pear, 1/2 cup blueberries)
- **Cooking Time:** 5 minutes

Homemade Low-Sodium Hummus

- **Ingredients:** 1 can chickpeas (rinsed and drained), 2 tablespoons tahini, 1 garlic clove, 2 tablespoons lemon juice, 2 tablespoons olive oil
- **Instructions:** Blend all ingredients until smooth. Serve with vegetable sticks.
- **Nutritional Information:** Calories: 180, Potassium: 250 mg, Sodium: 50 mg, Phosphorus: 90 mg
- **Serving Size:** 1/4 cup
- **Cooking Time:** 10 minutes

Desserts

Baked Apples

- **Ingredients:** 2 apples, cored and sliced, 1 tablespoon honey, 1/2 teaspoon cinnamon
- **Instructions:** Place apple slices in a baking dish. Drizzle with honey and sprinkle with cinnamon. Bake at 350°F for 20 minutes or until tender.
- **Nutritional Information:** Calories: 150, Potassium: 180 mg, Sodium: 0 mg, Phosphorus: 20 mg
- **Serving Size:** 1 apple
- **Cooking Time:** 25 minutes

Blueberry Muffins

- **Ingredients:** 1 cup all-purpose flour, 1/2 cup blueberries, 1/4 cup unsweetened applesauce, 1/4 cup honey, 1 teaspoon baking powder
- **Instructions:** Preheat oven to 350°F. Mix flour, baking powder, and blueberries in a bowl. Combine applesauce and honey, then mix with dry ingredients. Pour batter into muffin tin and bake for 20 minutes.
- **Nutritional Information:** Calories: 130, Potassium: 100 mg, Sodium: 10 mg, Phosphorus: 40 mg
- **Serving Size:** 1 muffin
- **Cooking Time:** 25 minutes

Conclusion

Navigating kidney disease requires a thoughtful approach to diet, as the foods we consume can have a profound impact on our health and well-being. Understanding the essential foods lists for kidney disease is crucial for anyone managing this condition. By adhering to these guidelines, individuals can effectively manage their symptoms, maintain optimal kidney function, and improve their overall quality of life.

Adhering to the recommended foods for kidney disease often means making significant changes to one's eating habits. Emphasizing low-potassium, low-phosphorus, and low-sodium options helps reduce the burden on the kidneys and prevent further deterioration. Fresh fruits, vegetables, lean proteins, and whole grains, when chosen carefully, can support kidney health while ensuring balanced nutrition.

On the other hand, avoiding certain foods is equally important. High-potassium and high-phosphorus foods can exacerbate kidney problems and lead to complications. Processed foods, which are often high in sodium, can also contribute to increased blood pressure and fluid retention, further stressing the kidneys. By steering clear of these foods, individuals can better manage their condition and avoid additional health issues.

Incorporating kidney-friendly recipes into daily meals can make managing the diet more manageable and enjoyable. Recipes that focus on fresh ingredients, appropriate seasoning, and balanced nutrition provide variety and satisfaction without compromising health. From breakfast options to snacks and desserts, there are numerous ways to create flavorful and nutritious meals that align with kidney dietary needs.

Regular monitoring and consultation with healthcare professionals are essential for tailoring dietary choices to individual health requirements. Personal needs may vary based on the stage of kidney disease, other health conditions, and treatment plans. Ongoing adjustments and professional guidance ensure that dietary strategies remain effective and responsive to changing health conditions.

Maintaining a kidney-friendly diet involves a combination of knowledge, planning, and flexibility. By understanding which foods support kidney health and which should be avoided, individuals can make informed choices that promote long-term well-being. The essential foods lists serve as a valuable tool in this journey, providing clear guidance and practical advice.

Ultimately, embracing the dietary recommendations in the essential foods lists for kidney disease empowers individuals to take control of their health. With careful planning and a focus on appropriate nutrition, it is possible to manage kidney disease

effectively and lead a fulfilling life. By prioritizing kidney health
through thoughtful food choices, individuals can enhance their
quality of life and achieve better health outcomes.